Prosopagnosia / Face Blindness Explained.

Prosopagnosia Types, Tests, Symptoms, Causes, Treatment, Research and Face Recognition all covered.

by

Lyndsay Leatherdale

Christmas 2015 .

All is revealed !!

With love,
Lyndyloo xxx

Published by IMB Publishing 2013

Table of Contents

Table Of Contents

Scope of this book

This book is designed to provide information on the condition of prosopagnosia or 'face blindness'. It will be of use to those who may benefit from gaining further information regarding this condition, whether it is for personal reasons, or to gain more of a general insight to the condition. It will cover the condition in terms of the general description, and also more specifically in terms of the subtypes that are currently identified. By doing this it will explicitly identify the similarities and differences between various types and degrees of prosopagnosia. In addition, this book will highlight some general theory behind the various causes of the condition, including research and case studies documented by various individuals internationally. The most up-to-date and current issues within research in prosopagnosia will also be highlighted within this text. We also come up to date in this book with a description of the current testing methods available to those who wish to be tested. As well as resources in order to help you, the individual, this book also contains general and relevant resources, both online and offline, which are suitable for those who are interested in learning more about this condition, with or without intent on using it for application.

This book is not designed to be a substitute for medical literature, however, it is a guide produced using material from reliable resources in order to gain a picture of how we understand, test for and treat prosopagnosia today.

Introduction

Would you be able to identify prosopagnosia if you came across it today? It is likely that you have heard someone tell you that they are terrible at recognising faces, but for many of us the term "prosopagnosia" would not be an immediate thought as the cause. Prosopagnosia, or "face blindness" is a disorder where an individual either has an impaired ability to recognise a face of someone who should be instantly recognisable, such as a friend or a family member (associative prosopagnosia), or more severely, they simply cannot see the form of the face clearly (apperceptive prosopagnosia). Despite face blindness or "prosopagnosia" being recognised since 1947, many of us are still very much in the dark about the condition. In recent years, we have learnt that prosopagnosia is a lot more common than previously thought. Studies are now showing an estimated 2.5% may be suffering from the condition, which includes cases where individuals acquired it from brain damage, and in most cases, those who have had the condition from birth via genetics.

As statistics are finally revealing the truth about the prevalence of this condition, it also reveals the other fact that many individuals in previous generations have been suffering from prosopagnosia without a medical diagnosis. Today, there exist various tests and some treatments available; however, there is still a lack of general awareness of prosopagnosia, which means that the condition is still affecting the lives of individuals who are simply unaware of the support and treatments available to them. As research develops and awareness grows, hope is that this will change in this current age.

Chapter 1) What is prosopagnosia?

According to the Oxford Dictionary, prosopagnosia is defined as *"The inability to recognize the faces of familiar people, typically as a result of damage to the brain."* This condition is also commonly known as 'face blindness' or 'facial agnosia'. Face blindness comes in various forms, so the way the condition can present itself can vary. Prosopagnosia can be present from birth, or it may arise suddenly as a result of brain damage such as brain trauma, stroke or neurodegenerative diseases. The way the condition can manifest also depends on the type and severity of the condition. As the condition is specific to faces, being face blind does not automatically mean that other visual processes, such as viewing objects in a scene, will be impaired. The fact that those suffering with prosopagnosia can quite easily identify other objects, means that they often use other cues in the environment to help identify individuals. For example an individual with prosopagnosia may use distinctive facial hair, jewellery, or a unique hairstyle as a cue. The treatment approach may also depend on the type and severity of the condition. A severe case would be a form where the patient is unable to see a face clearly in order to distinguish one face from another (apperceptive prosopagnosia), where a milder form would be that the patient cannot identify the individual, but can distinguish the face as unique (associative prosopagnosia). Prosopagnosia can be contrasted with visual agnosia. Visual agnosia is the deficit towards recognising objects by sight. The notion that both objects and facial deficits can occur separately gives us clues to how the visual system works. In terms of prosopagnosia research, this can help us towards a better understanding of this disorder. One of the main questions scientists face today is finding out if the deficit mechanism in prosopagnosia is exclusive for faces, or if there are other symptoms present in each case making prosopagnosia part of a more general visual deficit disorder. If prosopagnosia is indeed subject to faces only, we can answer the big question to whether specific mechanisms do exist within the brain to handle information for the face only.

1) Statistics for prosopagnosia

It has really just been within the last 10 years that claims came about that prosopagnosia is a widespread condition. Before this, prosopagnosia appeared in literature as a rare and isolated condition. The figure that currently repeatedly appears in reports, is 2.5% of the population who may have the disorder today. This percentage is thought to be predominantly those who suffer from congenital prosopagnosia, i.e. developmental prosopagnosia, which is inherited and present from birth.

The paper by medical researcher Ingo Kennerknecht in 2006, titled "First report of prevalence of non-syndrome hereditary prosopagnosia" revealed this statistic. Kennerknecht conducted a study on both medical personnel and school children. The study included 689 middle school pupils and found that 2.5% of his samples were identified to be sufferers of congenital prosopagnosia. These school children were not living their lives as though they were sufferers, but appeared to be going about their normal lives as though their condition wasn't there.

In 2008, in the paper "Neural and genetic foundations of face recognition and prosopagnosia", statistics were again depicting that prosopagnosia may affect around 2.5% of the German population. This research was conducted by medical doctors Grüter and his wife. These findings came up as quite astonishing at the time and Grüter was quoted to have said:

"So it's millions of people suffering from that, but it wasn't known,"

Grüter added that it's reasonable that the same would hold across Europe. From this data, it is often reported that generally we can decipher that approximately 2.5% of the general population may suffer from the condition.

It is clear from these studies that 2.5% is a good estimate of prosopagnosia in the population today. It is also clear that there is a range of severity to the condition. Whilst many of the isolated cases reported in the earlier documentation of prosopagnosia were more severe cases, these more recent studies give evidence that prosopagnosia does not necessarily mean that the case would need to be as severe as to interfere with everyday life. Research continues to support these statistics.

2) Defining face blindness

In 1937 Hoff and Pötzl suggested that face blindness should be considered as a specific type of visual agnosia. Ten years after this suggestion, Bodamer was the first to finally define the condition.

Joachim Bodamer was a German neurologist and a psychiatrist who worked at the Psychiatric Department Winnental in Winnenden. He produced various papers within psychiatry and brain diseases throughout his career and in 1947 Bodamer wrote a paper called "Die Prosop-Agnosie". These are classic Greek terms which literally translate into "face" and "non-knowledge". It was in this paper that the literature was presented with the term "Prosopagnosia" for the very first time. In this paper, Bodamer presented three cases, two of which had prosopagnosia. The individuals were German soldiers who acquired injuries during World War II. These observations were unique, as isolated cases previously appeared in the literature. Here we can see two patients side by side, suffering from face blindness. Moreover, Bodamer made it clear within the paper that there were no other problems with other aspects of their vision, such as viewing objects. This was enough for this paper to spark discussion that there may be specific facial mechanisms to recognise and perceive faces that were disturbed within these patients. Bodamer built up a strong case for a specific facial agnosia condition in this paper. The distinct display of symptoms gave a good and clear picture of what prosopagnosia was, and how the symptoms may be expressed. It also became apparent, even at this stage, that this was not a clear cut disorder and that it was comprised of various degrees of severity and manifestations. For example, one patient was unable to recognise faces, while another suffered with a distortion of facial perception. Symptoms were also not consistent as one of his patients was able to recognise faces in one moment, then unable to in the next.

The following are taken from Bodamer's text, which describes one of the cases observed.

"CASE 1: On 11.9.44 S went into a special hospital for brain injuries. After the injury, S was completely blind for several weeks. His sight returned gradually, in defined phases, but all impression of colour was missing – he could distinguish only light and dark, black and white...He said he had had difficulties with objects for a long time after his injury but he gradually got

14

to know objects again – he made mistakes now only with those objects he had not seen since his injury.

Also S had a disorder of the recognition of faces and, in a wider sense, of expressions... He could identify all the features of a face, but all faces appeared equally 'sober' and 'tasteless' to him...

25.11.44 S is told to look at his own face in the mirror. At first, he mistakes it for a picture but corrects himself. He stares for a long time, as though a totally strange object is before him, then reports he sees a face and describes its individual features...30.12.44. A picture of a long-haired dog, from the front, sitting [is shown]: S identifies it as human but with 'funny' hair." Bodamer (1947) as translated in Ellis and Florence 1990.

Researchers were very responsive to Bodamer's observations and for the next 20 years following this paper, a total of 70 papers reported cases of the disorder. This was an immensely sharp leap towards developing a better understanding of face blindness.

What has become apparent from subsequent studies is that there are two types of prosopagnosia. One of these was a facial recognition problem, and the other was a facial perception problem. These two different problems are now called associative and apperceptive prosopagnosia. There is also the third category of prosopagnosia, called "developmental prosopagnosia", which is prosopagnosia present at birth. Hence, we can now decipher prosopagnosia as both arising from injury, disease and also arising through genetic predisposition.

Chapter 2) The history of prosopagnosia

Whilst prosopagnosia is thought to have been prevalent throughout history, it was not actually defined as a condition until 1947. The first mention of face blindness symptoms within scientific literature can be dated back over a century prior to this by Arthur Wigan in 1844. Wigan was a medical practitioner who took an interest in face blindness and it is clear to us today that what was being observed in his work was indeed prosopagnosia. The following extract from one of his case studies exemplifies this.

"A gentleman of middle age, or a little past that period, lamented to me his utter inability to remember faces. He would converse with a person for an hour, but after an interval or a day, could not recognise him again. Even friends, with whom he has been engaged in business transactions, he was unconscious of ever having seen... When I inquire more fully into the matter, I found that there was no defect in vision, except that his eyes were weak, and that any long continued employment of them gave him pain. He was quite determined to conceal it, if possible, and it was impossible to convince him that it did not depend solely on the eyes. Wigan, A. L (1844). A new view of insanity: The duality of the mind.

Unlike later papers of the condition, the works by Wigan and a few other texts from the 19th century did not create a huge spark for many other researchers to explore these face blind symptoms further. This is evident in a 1987 paper by Quaglino & Borelli. One of the researchers, Antonio Quaglino was a professor of ophthalmology at Pavia, whilst Giambattista Borelli was a practising ophthalmologist in Turin. The paper they wrote was titled *"Loss of memory of the configuration of objects"*, which was written 22 years after the Wigan paper. In this paper, face blindness is still not described as a condition, which warrants classification. The observations seen in this paper were made on a 54 year old stroke patient who could no longer recognise faces. It is clearly demonstrated in the following passage that the symptoms portrayed are that of a patient with prosopagnosia:

"The patient no longer recognizes the faces of people, even those familiar to him at home and he has lost his orientation. During the first year he still retained the memory of figures of certain people and he could recall them by listening to their voices. However, for some time now he cannot remember them at all. He sees the figure as in a photograph, but less clearly....."

Despite the clear symptoms of prosopagnosia seen here, it wasn't until a whole 80 years after Quaglino & Borelli had written this paper that a term was finally coined by Joachim Bodamer.

Chapter 3) Subtypes of Prosopagnosia

There now exist various types of prosopagnosia. Apperceptive prosopagnosia is the inability to perceive faces. There is also associative prosopagnosia. This is the inability to recognise faces, whilst the individual can still perceive the face. There is also developmental prosopagnosia. This is where the individual has had prosopagnosia from birth.

1) Apperceptive prosopagnosia

Apperceptive prosopagnosia is the deficit of face processing. This means that those who suffer with this type of prosopagnosia are unable to see the facial features of the face, which we use to distinguish a particular face as different and unique from other faces. A practical example would be an individual who is presented with various photographs of faces. From this array of faces, an individual with apperceptive prosopagnosia will not be able to decipher whether the photos are of individuals who are the same, or different from each other. If the individual has a distinctive hairstyle or other characteristic features, this may provide a cue; however, going by facial processing alone, this wouldn't be possible. It is thought that the system affected in facial processing within apperceptive prosopagnosia is one of the earliest processes in face perception.

Here are some real life examples of individuals who present symptoms of apperceptive prosopagnosia.

Case Study 1

This case study was taken from the hugely popular book called *"The man who mistook his wife for a hat and other clinical tales"*. This book was written by neurologist Oliver Sacks in 1986. Sacks describes some of the patients he has come across in the past. One case study describes apperceptive prosopagnosia. The following was taken directly from the book, which describes the behaviour of someone with this condition as observed by Sacks.

"[He] started to look round for his hat. He reached out his hand, and took hold of his wife's head, tried to lift it off, to put it on. He has apparently mistaken his wife for a hat! His wife looked as if she was used to such things."

When Sacks observed the individual further he found that his apparent inability to recognise his wife was actually an inability to recognise faces in general. The following demonstrates how the individual was unable to follow the characters in a film.

"I turned on the television and found an early Bette Davis film. A love scene was in progress. Dr P. failed to identify the actress –

but this could have been because she had never entered his world. What was more striking was that he failed to identify the expressions on her face or her partner's, though in the course of a single torrid scene these passed from sultry yearning through passion, surprise, disgust and fury to a melting reconciliation. Dr P. could make nothing of any of this. He was very unclear as to what was going on, or who was who or even what sex they were. His comments on the scene were positively Martian."

Individuals suffering from apperceptive prosopagnosia are unable to recognise close family and friends as well as famous individuals unless there are other cues as shown in further text from this case below:

"On the walls of the apartment there were photographs of his family, his colleagues, his pupils, himself... By and large, he recognised nobody: neither his family, nor his colleagues, nor his pupils, nor himself. He recognised a portrait of Einstein, because he picked up the characteristic hair and moustache; and the same thing happened with one or two other people. 'Ach, Paul!' he said, when shown a portrait of his brother. 'That square jaw, those big teeth, I would know Paul anywhere!' But was it Paul he recognised, or one or two of his features, on the basis of which he could make a reasonable guess as to the subject's identity?"

Prosopagnosia can affect the memory of faces, even before the acquired injury as shown in the same case below:

"It was also evident that visual memories of people, even from long before the accident, were severely impaired – there was memory of conduct, or perhaps a mannerism, but not of visual appearance or face. Similarly, it appeared, when he was questioned closely, that he no longer had visual images in his dreams. Thus, as with Dr P, it was not just visual perception, but visual imagination and memory, the fundamental powers of visual representation, which were essentially damaged in this patient – at least those powers insofar as they pertained to the personal, the familiar, the concrete."

It is clear from this case that the patient was suffering from apperceptive prosopagnosia. The way which apperceptive prosopagnosia manifests can surface in different ways, as shown in Bodamer's case study of prosopagnosia in his 1947 paper.

Case study 2

In Bodamer's 1947 paper on prosopagnosia he describes a patient who would today be diagnosed with the subtype apperceptive prosopagnosia. This patient was a soldier who had suffered a bullet wound to the brain. When it came to looking at human faces, he described them as all looking the same.

"All faces appeared equally 'sober' and 'tasteless' to him..."
Bodamer (1947) as translated in Ellis and Florence 1990.

When he looked at a face he described them all as flat white ovals with dark eyes. He couldn't interpret facial expressions, although he could see movements of the face. Moreover, he was not able to identify his own face in the mirror. It is clear from this case study that the individual was suffering with apperceptive prosopagnosia.

Another of Bodamer's patients can be described in the next section as suffering from apperceptive prosopagnosia also. The following case study also provides good evidence that facial processing can be affected without affecting facial recognition. In this next case, one of the definitive statements which we can use to attribute their condition to apperceptive prosopagnosia is that they saw a face as distorted, with one eyebrow and the nose askew and the hair like an ill-fitting cap.

Case study 3

Bodamer's third case was different from the first two. A month after his injury he reported that all faces, including his own, were distorted in one way or another, for example the mouth was squint, one eyebrow was too high, or the nose was turned several degrees. This symptom was present for around 8 days. Despite this, the individual was still able to recognise an individual's face every time. Apart from viewing faces as skewed, the rest of the world appeared normal. It has subsequently been found that in similar cases reported, associative prosopagnosia doesn't usually accompany apperceptive prosopagnosia in the cases where facial features are distorted in this way.

We can see from the examples above that whilst it is clear that those suffering with apperceptive prosopagnosia are experiencing problems with their facial processing system, the way in which the deficit manifests varies greatly. From "hollowed out eyes" to "askew facial features" it seems that the way that the facial processing system is disrupted can vary. It is clear therefore that the way apperceptive prosopagnosia can manifest between individuals is wide.

2) Associative prosopagnosia

Associative prosopagnosia is, in a way, less severe, as the actual facial processing system is persevered in order for them to see the face. The problem is that they cannot attach an identity to faces. It is thought that this may be due to some disconnection between facial perception and their memory stores. In other cases, the memory of faces may be lost. With associative prosopagnosia, an individual may not be able to tell the difference between faces of their own friends and family.

Case studies for associative prosopagnosia

Case Study 1

In a paper by Tippett, published in 2000, an individual is described who has apperceptive prosopagnosia. The individual was aged 22 when he had a motorcycle accident. The patient then had an operation age 28 to remove his temporal cortex in order to alleviate his epilepsy. After the operation, he was unable to recognise hospital staff, or some members of his family. He was able to identify his wife only by her gait and hair only. He was also unable to remember any new faces after the operation. This was tested via a test that asked the patient to identify famous people who had risen to fame after the year of his operation. In this task he was able to identify 20/23 of the individuals who were famous before his operation, and only 8/17 of the individuals who became famous after. Moreover, it was his ability to specifically remember faces that had become impaired, whilst the ability to learn other visual stimuli remained intact.

Case study 2

Another case study that has highlighted how early brain damage can permanently affect the perception of faces was observed by Farah. Farah's patient was a 16 year old boy called Adam. At just one day old, he developed streptococcal meningitis. At the age of 6 it was visible to see lesions in the occipital and temporal cortices in both hemispheres. Whilst he had no symptoms of visual agnosia, he did have symptoms of prosopagnosia. When given the task to identify photos of famous individuals from non famous individuals, he was unable to identify a single famous face.

Case study 3

This next case study is of a 49 year old male who suffered with viral encephalitis. It took the patient one month to recover, however, he had now become prosopagnosic. He complained of not being able to recognise people's faces, especially if he met them after the disease. As is common with those with associative prosopagnosia, his ability to recognise individuals within context, were better than out of context. When an MRI and CT scan was taken, it showed that he suffered a lesion to the right temporal lobe.

3) Developmental prosopagnosia

Developmental prosopagnosia isn't another form of prosopagnosia in terms of symptoms; however, it does describe the origin of the disorder. Individuals with developmental prosopagnosia appear to suffer with the condition as a result of a genetic element or as a result of lesions before birth. The following is an example of developmental prosopagnosia, which is considered to make up the majority of those individuals who are said to suffer with the condition today.

Case study 1

In this case study, a 5 year old child who was born via a very normal pregnancy and completely normal development was reporting that he could not distinguish between faces. Whilst his ability to distinguish between faces was impaired, other aspects of his intellectual ability were developed. His reading ability was developing rapidly, as was his vocabulary. The child also has no family history of neurological or psychological problems. Whilst many of his intellectual abilities were positive, he frequently reported being lost. He was also spotted asking strangers if they were his friend, teacher or even mother or father. From these symptoms we can see that the child had developmental prosopagnosia. Without any brain damage or disease, this disorder seems to have a genetic element in this case.

Case study 2

This next case is a personal account written by an individual called Bill who has developmental prosopagnosia. Bill is fortunate enough to not only recognise his condition, but to become knowledgeable about what it means to have prosopagnosia:

"I was born with a condition that makes it difficult for me to recognize faces. There is a small part of the brain that is dedicated to that job, and though it is small, when it comes to recognizing faces, it is very very good. In me, that part doesn't work, making me blind to all but the most familiar of faces."

Bill describes how his condition has affected him on a particular occasion:

"Another time I was on a hike with about twenty guys. The group spread out along a trail, and I talked for about half an hour with a guy in blue jeans. We parted, and after about 15 minutes I began talking to a guy in red shorts. When I started the conversation with the usual introductory questions, he gave me a strange look and said we had just talked before. I denied having ever seen him before, and mentioned not having talked to anyone in red shorts. He said it had gotten warmer and he has ducked into some bushes to change. Then he recited back lots of the stuff we had talked about half an hour before."

This is a typical case of associative prosopagnosia.

The above shows cases of prosopagnosia that describe individuals who clearly have a particular subtype of prosopagnosia. Whilst it may be the case that each of these individuals did have a subtype of the condition, there are also cases where an individual may be suffering from more than one type. For example, someone with associative prosopagnosia, often comes with some symptoms of apperceptive prosopagnosia.

Chapter 4) Who gets it and why?

A lot has happened since the disorder was defined in 1947. We now have a huge amount of case studies within the literature, which have helped us to understand the disorder a great deal more since the term was first coined. The earliest cases reported tended to describe individuals who had severe cases of the disorder, which usually resulted from brain damage. We now know that there are milder forms, many of which exist from birth. The causes of prosopagnosia can be subdivided into categories. Prosopagnosia that has been acquired in someone who has previously had normal visual processing systems for recognising and processing faces is called "acquired prosopagnosia". There is also "congenital prosopagnosia", which is where prosopagnosia has arisen due to a genetic component. The three types of prosopagnosia previously mentioned include apperceptive (face processing deficit), associative (face recognition deficit) and developmental prosopagnosia. Developmental prosopagnosia can either be acquired, or congenital. It can be congenital if the condition was present due to genetic means, or it can be acquired if for example a lesion occurred in the brain before birth. A more in depth description of acquired and congenital prosopagnosia is given in the next section.

1) Congenital prosopagnosia

Congenital prosopagnosia is apparent face blindness from birth and is the most common form of prosopagnosia. This type of prosopagnosia can often be found to run in families. There are various case studies, which document this occurrence. This includes a study by Duchaine, Germine and Nakayama.

Case study 1

A study was conducted to include testing for 10 family members who may be suffering with prosopagnosia. This included 7 siblings, their mother and father, plus a maternal uncle. These individuals were all highly functioning in their lives. The family reported that they all had difficulties in recognising faces and that there were multiple incidents where facial recognition did not occur within the family, which also included the recognition of their own face in photographs or the mirror. The family has no history of potential sources of brain damage including head trauma or complications at birth.

Initial testing was done face to face, however, follow up tests were conducted remotely. When it came to testing for facial recognition, all members attained a low score. In addition, these members also attained a low score in object memory tasks. Therefore, this case gives an example where the ability to remember other object classes are also impaired.

Cases that demonstrate congenital prosopagnosia will also depict that the individuals have intact intellectual and sensory function and there is no neurological evidence to suggest that damage has caused the symptoms. Whilst tests show that many individuals test positive for this disorder, the specific genes responsible for prosopagnosia are yet to be discovered. Moreover, how these genes may be involved within the neuropsychological mechanisms in face blindness are also yet to be found.

2) Acquired prosopagnosia

Acquired prosopagnosia is face blindness that has developed with an individual who has not experienced face blindness previously. This type of prosopagnosia may originate from a head injury, stroke or degenerative diseases. Some of the cases mentioned in Chapter 3 are those who have acquired prosopagnosia. Despite there being cases where it appears that the individual who has acquired prosopagnosia has no aphasia for object recognition, some researchers do not fully accept this as being true. If indeed those who have acquired prosopagnosia have no other visual aphasia other than for faces, it gives us good evidence that facial processing is ran via domain specific mechanisms. Cases observing patients who have acquired prosopagnosia are quite important as this form is very rare.

Chapter 5) Neural basis for prosopagnosia

There has been a lot of research surrounding the neural basis for prosopagnosia. A lot of research has accumulated evidence that suggest that the fusiform face area may hold the key for facial processing, and therefore prosopagnosia.

1) Fusiform Face Area (FFA)

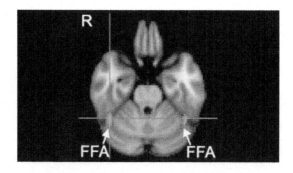

Fusiform Face Area. Image source: http://www.brainfacts.org

The fusiform face area is a portion of the visual system, which is thought to potentially be specialized for facial recognition. The FFA is located in the fusiform gyrus area. There is now evidence to suggest that certain abnormalities in the FFA area of the brain may be linked to prosopagnosia. Research currently continues to investigate

34

whether this is true. There have been various studies using PET and fMRI that show us that the fusiform gyrus area of the brain is linked to the visual processing of faces. For example, studies show that the right hemisphere is more active when subjects view faces, compared to when they view common non-face objects. This region of the brain is also more active during face matching tasks in comparison to the viewing of scrambled faces, location matching, letter strings, or textures. Despite there being a large correlation of prosopagnosic patients who don't shown activity in this area, there has also been studies of individuals who do not have prosopagnosia, who have shown to have the same result as those with prosopagnosia in the FFA area. Therefore scientists cannot be certain that this correlation exists. In addition, there have also been other face selective regions which have been identified to disrupt facial processing which include: ventral occipital cortex, the superior temporal sulcus, and it has been shown that the anterior potion of these areas can lead to deficits in face processing, including prosopagnosia.

2) Face specific neurons

Whilst we can see from the studies on the FFA that we know which part of the brain is most active in facial recognition tasks, as mentioned previously, the biggest question in this field is discovering if there are face specific areas, which are exclusively for the face, or if these areas are used for more general visual processing, of which facial processing falls into its category. A more specific question probed by researchers is if there are truly mechanisms that are face specific. One angle of research this has been investigated by is the observations of facial neurons. Do neurons exist that are specific to the viewing of the face? Research suggests that this may be the case.

There is a lot of research about visual specific neurons. For example, researchers have found that there are neurons that are tuned to respond to 'bars' only – but how about faces? Faces are a lot more complex than bars, and for this reason a lot of researchers are reluctant to firmly speculate that there are neurons which respond exclusive to faces. Despite this reluctance, many cases do support that there is evidence to show that there may exist face specific neurons. Research continues in this area.

We can see here that there are two main causes for prosopagnosia; one genetic cause; the other cause being acquired cases. So therefore, the people who get this disorder either have a genetic predisposition (which is dominant), or they acquire it completely through unfortunate circumstances, such as brain damage. If an individual suspects they may have prosopagnosia, either as a result of an acquired route, or if they suspect they might have it via genetic means – what signs can they look out for? Typical signs and symptoms are explained in the next section.

Chapter 6) Symptoms of prosopagnosia

It's not uncommon to hear someone say that they have trouble in recognising faces. You may even experience it yourself from time to time without having the condition prosopagnosia. However, if you are diagnosed with the condition, and you know someone else who has it, you may find that there are common symptoms which are prevent with this condition. So what are the general symptoms of someone who has prosopagnosia? The Yahoo Face blind group is a well established online group who have worked together to compile the following list of 7 common signs of prosopagnosia. An individual with face blindness may identify with some, or all of the following symptoms.

Failing to recognise close friends or family members in unexpected situations

Many case studies of prosopagnosia show that being unable to recognise close family or friends outside of context is one sign of the condition. This means family and friends that may be more easily recognised at home, at school, or at work than in environments out of context - for example at a gym. It is for this reason that you will often find that these individuals will try very hard to use other cues, such as a distinctive hairstyle for example, to remember the individual. This leads on to the next symptom.

When meeting someone new, you remember something distinctive about that individual such as a hairstyle or a distinctive features rather than their face.

Many cases of prosopagnosia mention that the individual develops specific coping mechanisms in order to deal with their condition. These coping mechanisms are usually visual cues, which are distinctive and can be explicitly associated with a specific individual so that they can be identified. Other cues may be used, which are not visual, such as using their voice for example, as a cue. Helping patients enhance their use of other visual cues is actually a way in which treatment is currently provided. Without doing this, many prosopagnosic sufferers would be at a loss on how to distinguish individuals.

Trouble in following films or television shows that have more than a few distinctive characters.

Prosopagnosia means that there may be trouble with not only identifying people who should be familiar, such as friends and family, but also famous people on screen. This also includes any new characters, which might need to be quickly learned in order to get involved in the plot. This will be very difficult for someone with prosopagnosia, especially if the characters do not have a very distinctive look.

Failing to recognize yourself in the mirror and/or have difficulty identifying yourself in photographs.

Suffering with prosopagnosia does not only mean that you will have difficulty recognizing the familiar people in your life, but it also means that you may have difficulty recognizing your own face.

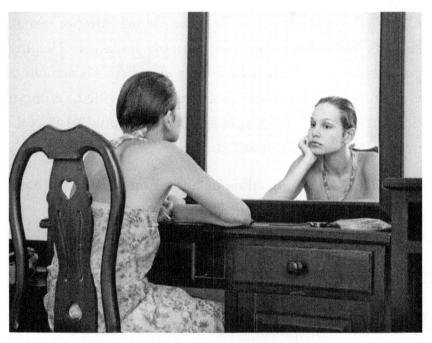

A common symptom of prosopagnosia is being unable to recognise your own reflection.

When someone casually waves or says hello in the street, you more often than not don't know who they are.

Walking down the street and saying hello to someone that you know, is a normal thing for someone without the condition of prosopagnosia. However, there are those with prosopagnosia who would find this situation embarrassing and quite a lot of the time will try to avoid these situations. There are reports that ways to deal with this have been to cross over the road, for example, so that there is no confrontation or embarrassment of what they know is inevitably going to happen.

When someone gets a haircut, you may not recognize them when you see them again.

Those with prosopagnosia often develop coping mechanisms, which are used in everyday life to distinguish one person from another. This may be cues, such as jewellery or tattoos, for example. Another example would be hairstyles. An individual who has a distinctive hairstyle will be recognized better than someone who has a regular hairstyle. This means that if someone with prosopagnosia is using hair as a cue for recognition, and that individual gets a haircut, then this cue will disappear. This will often mean that they no longer have enough information to identify that individual.

You have difficulty recognizing neighbours, friends, co-workers, clients, schoolmates etc, out of context.

Another common symptom those with prosopagnosia experience is that they are more likely to not be aware that their close friends or family are in the same area if they are in a context that is not of their usual nature. For school friends, this would be at school, for brothers and sisters, this would be at home, or a work co-worker, this would be in the work environment. People with prosopagnosia will find it difficult to identify individuals who are not in their usual locations. For example, a school friend at a football match, or a work college at a school play. In these situations, an individual with prosopagnosia may not even realize that their loved ones are in the same area.

In addition to the symptoms compiled by the Yahoo group, there are also other signs of the condition:

- **Lack of navigation skills** - Those with prosopagnosia often find it difficult to navigate. For this reason, these individuals are prone to getting lost.

- **Inability to recognise emotions** – Those with associative prosopagnosia may have the inability to recognise faces. It is often also the case that they are unable to identify the emotion of the individual as well.

- **Inability to recognise left from right** – This is another symptom, which is often reported in those who suffer from prosopagnosia.

- **Inability to identify race or colour** – It may not only be the case that individuals with prosopagnosia cannot identify the individual, but recognising the race and/ or colour of the individual may prove difficult.

- **Difficulty in reading literature** – It may be difficult for an individual to follow a story in a book. This is due to the fact that an individual has difficulty in imagining the faces of the characters described in the book.

More likely to develop in males than females?

One observation has been that prosopagnosia is more prevalent in males than females. It is thought however, that this is a reflection of the higher number of strokes that occur in males than in females. Therefore, subsequently, there will be a higher number of males who will potentially suffer from prosopagnosia as a result.

It may be difficult to monitor your own symptoms of prosopagnosia, whether you are a school student, or a housewife, or even a celebrity. There are many notable individuals who experience prosopagnosia, who are able to handle their disorder, and still be very successful.

Chapter 7) Notable individuals with prosopagnosia

As mentioned previously, this condition is actually considered to be highly prevalent in the population. Whilst many may go through their lives without a diagnosis, there will also be those individuals who have been fortunate enough to recognise their condition. Below describes some of the notable individuals who are known to have prosopagnosia. Some of these individuals are from the past, and there are some who still exist today.

Duncan Bannatyne

Duncan Bannatyne is an entrepreneur from Scotland. He has become a household name in recent years through the popular UK TV show Dragons' Den. Whilst in the show he offers to help other businesses succeed with help from his own business network; he has also been suffering with prosopagnosia. The world of business has many faces to remember, however, despite Duncan Bannatyne not having the skills to recognise faces, his strive for success and accomplishment has not been affected. Duncan Bannatyne talks about his condition and how he has coped with it in the past in the quote below:

"I remember as a child not recognising certain people and actually walking across the road because I thought do I know that person? Or don't I know that person? I didn't want to embarrass myself by walking past them, or saying hello to them if I didn't know them. The big incident that happened, was when I was here about 5-6 years ago and we had a board meeting where we met our new auditors and we spent about 3 -4 hours with them. I went home and that night we had a black tie do. So I was with my managing director and my wife and we were standing there, a crowd of us, this little chap came over and started talking to us and I started talking politely thinking, well he knows me and I don't know him and he went away and I said to my managing director Nigel Armstrong – who was that? He said that's your new auditor, we appointed him this morning and he laughed. I spent 4 hours in that guy's company and I cannot remember meeting him before."

As seen from this extract from an interview, he has often found in business that he has had to bluff his way through situations where his prosopagnosia may prevent him from remembering individuals in certain situations.

Despite gaining a huge amount of success in wealth, Duncan Bannatyne has admitted that at times, bluffing has not always worked and it has in the past affected his business relationships:

"I think it's probably affected my career in the form of business relationships, because I don't really have any great business relationships! There was a little incident, which I thought was quite crazy...I was in the portacabin and a bloke came in who was doing some photocopying and he started talking to me. After 10 minutes he said to me, 'You don't know who I am do you?' and I said, 'No' and he said 'I'm the manager of your Liverpool club.' He said 'You appointed me 3 days ago.' This made him very angry, and so he quit. I didn't realize he quit until about 3 or 4 days later when I was told that I'd upset him. I didn't realize I'd upset him, it's not my fault I didn't recognise him- it's as simple as that."

Robert Cecil

Robert Cecil, the leader of the conservative party in 1878, was thought to have suffered from prosopagnosia. His grandson David Cecil, wrote of the prosopagnosia symptoms in his book *"The Cecils of Hatfield House"*. The following passage was taken from this book where he writes about his grandfather's inability to recognise familiar faces.

"He found it hard to recognize his fellow men, even his relations, if he met them in unexpected circumstances. Once, standing behind the throne at a Court ceremony, he noticed a young man smiling at him. "Who is my young friend", he whispered to a neighbour. "Your eldest son", the neighbour replied... He was

also vague about people he did not know. Driving up from Hatfield station one evening he found himself in the company of a man who seemed to know him and whom he therefore took to be some unrecognised old acquaintance. Suddenly, the man spoke. 'Lord Sailsbury', he said in solemn tones, 'I am to bring you a message from almighty god.' My grandfather said nothing, but on his arrival went to his study, and sitting down to work, summoned a manservant. 'I have left a madman in the front hall,' he said calmly, 'could you see that he is got rid of' and returned to his papers."

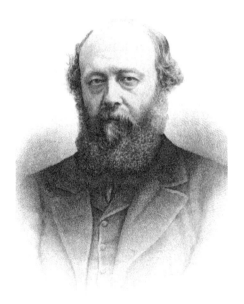

Robert Cecil suffered with prosopagnosia.

Chuck Close

The American painter and photographer is one of those individuals who you may think is the least likely of people to suffer from prosopagnosia. Chuck is known as the "reigning portraitist of the information age". While he might spend a lot of his time painting large-scale portraits, at the same time, in the real world, he has prosopagnosia and is unable recognise faces. He said that he was compelled to do portraits as a way to help him remember the important people in his life.

Chuck close also gave us some insight as to his coping mechanisms at the World Science Festival interview where he said the following about coping with the condition:

"My approach is to be more outgoing and more friendly and to try and charm my way through things. I also lecture and talk all the time about face blindness and my other problems, so that people are aware that I have them and cut me some slack. Self deprecating humour will cover it a great deal."

7

Jane Goodal

Jane Goodal is a British primatologist, anthropologist, ethologist and UN messenger of Peace. Jane is also now considered to be the world's foremost expert on chimpanzees. She is most well known for her 45 year study of social and family interactions of wild chimpanzees in Gombe Stream National Park, Tanzania. Jane mentions her prosopagnosia in her autobiography of which an excerpt is given below:

"In the course of my travels, one thing detracts from my enjoyment of meeting people. I suffer from an embarrassing, curiously humbling neurological condition called prosopagnosia, which, translated, means I have problems with face recognition. I used to think it was due to some mental laziness, and I tried desperately to memorize the faces of people I met so that, if I saw them the next day, I would recognize them. I had no trouble with those who had obvious physical characteristics – unusual bone structure, beaky nose, extreme beauty or the opposite. But with the other faces, I failed, miserably. Sometimes I knew that people were upset when I did not immediately recognise them – certainly I was. Because I was embarrassed, I kept it to myself. Quite by chance, when talking to a friend recently, I found that he suffered from the same problem. I could not believe it. Then I discovered my own sister, Judy, knew similar embarrassment. Perhaps others did, also. I wrote to the well-known neurologist Dr. Oliver Sacks. Had he ever heard of such an unusual condition? Not only had he

heard of it -- he suffered from it himself! His situation was far more extreme than mine. He sent me a paper, titled 'Developmental memory impairment: faces and patterns,' by Christine   Temple.

Even now that I know I need not feel guilty, it is still difficult to know how to cope -- I can hardly go around telling everyone I meet that I probably won't know them from Adam the next time I see them! Or maybe I should? It is humiliating, because most people simply think I'm making an elaborate excuse for my failure to recognize them and that, obviously, I don't really care about them at all -- so they are hurt. I have to cope as best I can -- usually by pretending to recognize everyone! While that can have its awkward moments too, it's not nearly as bad as the other way around."

Despite Jane clearly demonstrating that she does experience some difficulties with the condition, she has managed to carve herself a very successful and rewarding career.

Hubert Dreyfus

Hubert L Dreyfus is an American Philosopher. His major interests are phenomenology, existentialism, and philosophy of psychology, philosophy of literature and philosophical implications of artificial intelligence. Dreyfus is part of the Philosophy department at UC Berkeley College. The following can be found within his profile page from the college website which is designed to prepare his students for the inevitable lack of recognition their teacher has.

"Prof. Dreyfus suffers from a mild case of prosopagnosia or 'face blindness'. So, although he has met you before, and sometimes more than once, it is quite probable that he will not recognize you when you meet again. Please, re-introduce yourself telling him when and where you met the previous time(s). Thank you. "

Many individuals who suffer from prosopagnosia have tried various ways to prevent others from interpreting their condition as being rude. Dreyfus here has applied a subtle, yet very useful warning on his profile to prevent awkward situations.

Oliver Sacks

Oliver Sacks is a famous neuroscientist and author of many books, including *"The Man Who Mistook His Wife for a Hat"* which in fact includes observations from one of his patients who suffered from prosopagnosia. Oliver Sacks of course knows what prosopagnosia is, however it did not occur to him until middle age when people became shocked that he confused one of his brothers with the other, that he might suffer with the condition. Following discussing it with family members, he learned that a number of them had similar difficulties with face recognition also. The following is taken from his World science festival interview

"Usually my assistant Kate will say to people beforehand, before they come in -'Don't ask if he remembers you because he will say no.' To me she says, 'Don't just say no...say I am awful with faces, I wouldn't recognise my own mother.' I tend to withdraw....but it doesn't solve it, it often makes it worse."

Oliver Sacks has become known to talk about his condition on various occasions. An extract describing how the condition may mean he gets misrepresented at times with those who do not know he suffers with the condition can be found below:

"This has been life-long, and it has caused offense and embarrassment and bewilderment and I would have to apologize to people every day for forgetting them all. I thought I was, I think, inattentive or careless, and it was only later that I began to realize, especially when I met an older brother whom I hadn't seen for decades and he had exactly the same problem, that this might be some odd family thing, and if we had it in our family, it might be common elsewhere. When 'The Man Who Mistook His Wife For A Hat' book came out in 1986, I received, in fact I continue to receive, dozens of letters from people who spoke of lifelong difficulties recognising faces."

Brad Pitt

Brad Pitt is one of those figures in the entertainment industry, who is often praised for his looks, however despite him being in a world which has a large focus on aesthetics, he openly admits that he has difficulties in recognising faces. His condition became public knowledge with the interview which was conducted for Esquire magazine in the June/July issue of 2013. Pitt speaks about how his condition affects those around him:

"So many people hate me because they think I'm disrespecting them,"

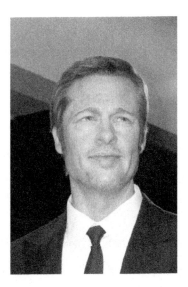

Brad Pitt famously claimed to have the condition in an interview conducted by Esquire magazine.

He admits to previously trying to cope with the condition by just asking individuals where he met them before, but he admits that this made things worse.

"People were more offended...Every now and then, someone will give me context, and I'll say, 'Thank you for helping me.' But I piss more people off. You get this thing, like, 'You're being egotistical. You're being conceited.' But it's a mystery to me, man. I can't grasp a face, and yet I come from such a design/aesthetic point of view."

Mary Ann Sieghart

Mary Ann Sieghart is currently a radio presenter and journalist. She was also a former assistant editor of The Times. Her topics of interest are lifestyle, social affairs and politics. Not only does Mary suffer from prosopagnosia, but her husband and daughter are also face blind. Mary has been quoted to have said the following about coping with the condition.

"It's a great source of social embarrassment, as I just can't remember if I know that person and if I do, where I might know them from..."

Her husband also shares her embarrassment of social situations as he speaks about hosting their own party.

"We've always been useless at parties and usually spend the whole evening whispering 'who was that?' to each other, so you can imagine how nervous we were holding our own....My daughter even joked that we should all have T-shirts saying 'Don't blame me, I'm prosopagnosic' to get us out of tricky social situations. "It's awful when people think you're being rude by not recognising them even though you might see them every day."

These notable individuals are just some of the individuals that we know about and no doubt there are more who may not even be aware that they have the condition. We can see here that prosopagnosia has affected all types of individuals: men, women, those with high artistic ability to those with high scientific ability. Prosopagnosia can affect anyone.

Chapter 8) Diagnosis and current testing methods for prosopagnosia

Diagnosis

Those who have the developmental kind of prosopagnosia from birth may find it very difficult to communicate exactly how the condition is affecting them. It may be especially difficult if they are not aware that the condition exists at all. A diagnosis is usually made as a result of a cognitive assessment. An individual may also be referred to a clinical neuropsychologist within the NHS (for the UK), or to a private practise.

Testing methods

There are some tests that are used within both research and as an individual testing means for diagnosis. These tests are widespread and are currently very good at identifying those with prosopagnosia. As we develop our knowledge of prosopagnosia, researchers are seeking to improve the way we test for prosopagnosia to ensure that the public get the best testing methods possible.

Testing for prosopagnosia may come in two parts – one for testing if there is a facial recognition problem (associative prosopagnosia), and the other is to test if it is a facial perception problem (apperceptive prosopagnosia).

1. Facial identification tasks are used to test if the individual has a facial recognition problem i.e. if they have associative prosopagnosia. A typical test would be a presentation of famous faces, and non famous faces. The task would be to distinguish the famous faces, from the non famous faces.

2. Face matching tasks are used to test if the individual has a facial perception problem i.e. apperceptive prosopagnosia. In this task, individuals are presented with the same face in different views and are to match them together.

The Warrington Recognition Memory Test for Faces (RMF) and the Benton Facial Recognition Test (BFRT) are both tests that are currently used by cognitive neuropsychologists and clinicians. The following describes both of these tests in more detail.

1) Warrington face recognition test

This is a facial recognition task; therefore it is specifically useful in determining if an individual is likely to have associative prosopagnosia. This was actually initially designed to test non-verbal memory without it being specific towards prosopagnosia. Over time, its use as a test for prosopagnosia became known. In this test, individuals are presented with 50 black and white photographs. One of these photographs will be presented every 3 seconds. In response to each photograph, the individual will state if the face is pleasant or unpleasant. The response "yes" will indicate that the face is pleasant, and the response "no" will indicate that the individual finds the face unpleasant. Once all of the faces have been presented to them, it is followed by another task. This next task will include some of the photos that they have previously seen, and some photos that they have not seen. Each photo will be presented in couples – one will be a face they have seen previously, and the other one will be a distracter photo. The task is to identify the photos that they have previously seen and so the task now becomes a task for memory. Individuals with associative prosopagnosia are not able to recognise the individuals that they have previously seen, i.e. they are not able to store a face in their memory. This test will exercise this ability, and therefore can be used to isolate individuals with the condition associative prosopagnosia. Once the test is complete, the number of correct choices determines the final score. The maximum score attainable from the test is the identification of 50 faces. The mean range is between 42.4 and 44.4, depending on the age group and the standard deviations of approx 3.5.

2) Benton face recognition test

This is a face processing task, so it is especially useful in determining if an individual is likely to have apperceptive prosopagnosia. Apperceptive prosopagnosia can be tested using this test, as it requires the individual to match faces from different angles and different lighting. As those with the condition cannot process faces, the ability to match faces would not be possible. There are two versions of the Benton Face Recognition Test that are available. One is considered as the short form, with 13 items and the other is considered the long form, containing 27 items. The way the Benton Face recognition test works is that the individual is first presented with a target photo. This photo will need to be viewed by the individual carefully in order to identify the same face from 6 other photos. There are 3 sections to this test, each slightly different. In the first of these tests the individual is required to match the frontal view of the target face, with another frontal photo (but not the exact same photograph) of the same individual. The next task is that the frontal view of the target face will need to be matched with another three photos of the same individual, but taken at various different angles. The final part of the test is that the individual needs to match the target face with 3 other photos of the target face, which were taken in different lighting conditions. We have seen in case studies that the inability to process faces in the apperceptive prosopagnosic can manifest in various ways. One individual viewed the features on a face as skewed and another saw faces as all the same, flat white shape with hollowed out eyes. What is consistent however, is their inability to view features as they really are. This test is good for picking up on these kinds of symptoms.

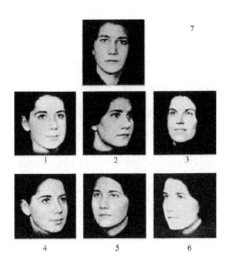

The Benton Face Recognition Test. The task is to match the photo at the top, with 3 of the photos at the bottom. (Image source: 'Duchaine, B. C, & Weidenfeld,A. (2003). An evaluation of two commonly used tests of unfamiliar face recognition. *Neuropsychologia'* 2002.)

Picture Source : www.faceblind.org

7

3) Possible improvements of current testing methods

Despite these tests being very useful, they do not go without criticism. The main issue is that these tests may not be designed in the best way to test for the recognition and visual process of the "features" of the face only. We know that a coping strategy that those with prosopagnosia use is to use cues, such as distinctive visual characteristics, to help them identify the individual. The problem here is that researchers say there is room for individuals to pass the test even if they have the disorder. This is due to the individual using other visual cues, other than facial features, to match the target photo. An example would be that features such as the eyebrows, could be used to discriminate between the target face and the distracter. This criticism has been found in the literature for both the Warrington face test, and the Benton facial recognition test. Researchers continually work to find the best possible testing methods for this condition. An improvement to these tests would be a new design approach, where hair would not be included in the photographs.

Chapter 9) Treatment

As prosopagnosia is a condition which can either be acquired, or inherited, the way in which we can look at recovery can therefore vary, depending on the type and severity of prosopagnosia the subject has.

For acquired prosopagnosia there is evidence to suggest that it is possible to recover. A study by Goldsmith and Liu in 2001 discovered that this recovery usually took around 9 weeks in total. Unfortunately, there is no current cure for developmental prosopagnosia. However, the therapies that do exist encourage the patient (for both types) to cope with the condition by using other cues within the environment to help identify individuals. These can be in the form of visual cues, or non visual cues. It must also be kept in mind that these techniques need to be sensitive to those who experience agnosia for classes of objects for example, or particular aspects of vision, such as line orientation, colour or luminance. These symptoms quite often accompany those with prosopagnosia. The following provides some of the cues that those with prosopagnosia may use, or may be taught to use as a coping mechanism for the condition.

Visual cues

These may include:

- **Jewellery** – An individual may be identified via their wedding band or distinctive facial and body piercings.
- **Clothing** – Distinctive clothing can be used as a cue. This is especially useful as an initial cue when first meeting people in social situations for short periods of time, such as parties and business meetings.
- **Facial Hair** – Facial hair, such as a distinctive moustache or beard, can be used as a cue.
- **Tattoos** – A unique tattoo may be used as a cue. Tattoos on parts of the body that are always exposed will provide the best cue for the individual with prosopagnosia. This includes tattoos on the hands, arms or neck area.
- **Weight** – An individual may have distinctive proportions, which may make them easy to recognise for a prosopagnosia sufferer.
- **Height** – An individual may have a distinctive height- so be very tall, or short for example. This will also help an individual with identification.
- **Hairstyle** – This is a common cue, which is often mentioned in the literature. A distinctive hairstyle can be effectively used as a cue to recognise

individuals. This will remain a cue until of course an individual decides to change their hairstyle.

- **Distinctive features** – It's often reported that extreme features have also been used to recognise individuals. Reports show that individuals who appear extremely beautiful, or not so attractive are more likely to be recognized by an individual with prosopagnosia, than those who are plain looking.
- **Gait** – This is the pattern of movement of the limbs, which may be used to help identify unique individuals. This will be especially useful if an individual has a distinctive gait.
- **Mannerisms** – Many of us have distinctive mannerisms, such as nervous ticks, which can be used to successfully identify an individual.
- **Possessions** – The individual you see regularly may always have a distinctive object with them, such as a walking stick, a particular bike or car, etc which can be used as cues.

As prosopagnosia does not usually affect other parts of the visual system other than faces, it is possible that these cues can be used with a high degree of success. As demonstrated in the various case studies throughout this book, using cues is something which has become very important to many of those suffering with the disorder.

Non visual cues

Whilst most of the cues will be visual, there are also non visual cues that may be used. These, however, may not provide such a quick reaction in comparison to visual cues.

- **Smell** – If an individual, for example, always wears the same perfume, this may also be an additional cue that those with prosopagnosia may be able to work with.

- **Voice** – Voices are very individual and distinctive and can be used to identify an individual from their tone or accent, for example.

The above cues can be used in therapies to help the individual to master the art of using these cues in everyday life. For some, it can make all the difference when it comes to social interaction.

Other useful coping strategies

In addition to using cues, patients with prosopagnosia have also helped to provide a list of other strategies (as provided by Headways), which can be used. These are provided below:

In social situations

Wait before calling someone by name – It is better to wait until you're 100% sure before calling someone by name to avoid any embarrassment.

Be friendly to everyone in social situations – Many of those with prosopagnosia will often say that having the disorder can make you appear rude or arrogant. To avoid this, a good strategy is to smile and be friendly to everyone in social situations.

Meet fewer people at one time – If you have the choice to have a gathering, choose fewer individuals, rather than many. Having many individuals around that you do not recognise at one time will be more difficult to manage than just a few.

Ask individuals of the opposite sex about the individual you are looking for - If you are looking for a male friend at a party, it is better to ask a group of women where he may be rather than a group of men. It may be the case that you end up asking the person you are looking for if you approach a group of the same sex.

Develop good conversational skills - Those with prosopagnosia may benefit from developing their conversational skills. This will not only help you to build confidence, but the more you take interest in individuals, the more information can be used as cues for future meetings.

Take a friend with you - If you are really apprehensive about going to a party, for example, and not recognising anyone, it is a good idea to bring a friend along with you.

This friend should ideally also have the same friends so will be able to assist you in identifying the people around you.

As this condition has recently been revealed to be a lot more common than previously thought, the demand for learning about potential treatments has increased. There are currently training programs in development, which aim to improve face recognition skills for those with prosopagnosia. These programs in development do not claim to be providing a cure for the condition, but for a means to improve their recognition skills, where possible.

From finding out you have prosopagnosia, to researching what the condition actually is, many of you may find that all of the questions have not yet been answered, and so there is still a lot of research taking place regarding facial processing. One of the ways researchers are moving forward with our facial processing knowledge is via creating models of how we process faces. A visual representation of face processing is the most simple way we can look at the facial processing system, so it is something which is useful not only for researchers, but for anyone who would like to learn more about face processing.

Chapter 10) How do we process faces?

Documenting how prosopagnosia can manifest helps scientists to build up a picture of how we process faces. It will also help scientists gain a better understanding of why the various symptoms of prosopagnosia occur. There are big questions to be answered in regards to face recognition and processing such as "Are there specific mechanisms to view faces and if so, what evidence shows this?" Previous chapters have reviewed some case studies, which have told us which part of the brain is disrupted in those who have prosopagnosia. It is these kinds of studies that will pave the way for a better understanding of facial processing in the future. What is considered to be our current optimal understanding of facial processing and recognition today? Which face models are considered to be our most true representation of faces? The following are a couple of the most highly regarded face models.

1) Bruce and Young's Model

One of the most widely accepted models that describes the stages in face processing was developed by Bruce and Young in 1986. The basis for this model is something that they called "viewed centred description". This was coined to describe the process where we create an internal structural model of the face. Once this model has been created, Bruce and Young say that this allows the individual to perform higher processing functions such as "facial recognition" and "facial differentiation". Individuals with apperceptive prosopagnosia cannot process the internal model of the face from looking at a face. This suggests that in these patients the "view centred description" process is disrupted. The higher processing function of "facial recognition" would be disrupted in an individual with associative prosopagnosia.

Evaluation of Bruce and Young's model

There are positive and negative aspects to this model. One of the main criticisms is that the model is quite vague. In particular, researchers have criticised the cognitive aspect of the model to be quite indistinct.

Despite this, however, this model is supported by various case studies. It also coincides with the way facial processing has been viewed in PET scans. Results from PET scans show that different areas of the brain are active when processing faces. This suggests that facial processing is a modular activity. This coincides with the modular way this model presents how we look at faces.

2) Valentine's Model

Valentine's model remains inspirational to research focussing on the relationship between different faces in memory. In this model, each face is represented as a point or a vector in a multidimensional space, or "face space". The multidimensional space has a number of dimensions of which each represent a parameter extracted from the face upon detection. Therefore, each point or vector in the multidimensional space is positioned depending on the properties of the parameters extracted from the face. Hence, the relationship between two faces in the multidimensional space is represented by two points or vectors, of which the distance between these two points or vectors is proportional to the degree of which the parameters of the two faces are similar.

Valentine used the multidimensional space framework to propose two kinds of models:

1) **Norm-based model (N-BC) :**

In the norm-based model, each face is represented as a vector distance from a norm representation of the face. The parameters of the norm representation, is the average of all the detected faces in the multidimensional space, which is

71

situated at the origin of the multidimensional space. Each face is represented by a vector line which begins at the origin and extends out into the multidimensional space proportional to how different the parameters of the detected face is from the parameters of the norm face at the origin. Therefore, the similarity between two faces is proportional to the distance between the vectors in the multidimensional space.

2) Exemplar-based model (PE-B):

In the exemplar-based model, each face is represented as a point in the multidimensional space. The position of this point depends on the properties of the parameters of the detected face. However, unlike the N-BC model, each face in the exemplar-based model is not represented by the degree of similarity to the parameters of the norm representation of the face at the origin. Instead, each face is its own independent absolute representation, being only relative to other faces in the multidimensional space. The degree of similarity between two faces is proportional to the distance between the two points in the multidimensional space.

Norm-based coding (N-BC) model and the b) Exemplar-based coding (PE-B) model.

a) **The N-BC model**   b)   **The PE-B model**

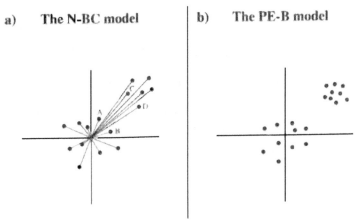

Visual representation of the N-BC model and the PE-B model
(Rokover et al, 2001)

Evaluation of Valentine

This model successfully explains various face processing observations. For example, it can explain why we can detect a typical face quicker than a distinctive face. Despite that this model can account for some observable properties of face processing, others criticise Valentine's model for being merely a basic metaphorical and visual representation of how faces relate to one another, without much consideration of the real mechanisms in face perception. For example, Valentine describes that the measure of similarity between two faces is the distance between two points in the multidimensional space. Hence, the distance between the two points represents the variations of the parameters in a face. Yet, in order to describe what the variation of parameters across the multidimensional space represent, we need to refer to the parameters which Valentine referred to in his description of the model.

Whilst these models hold promise for researchers today, there are still various criticisms. It is this kind of research that can potentially lead us towards gaining a better understanding of prosopagnosia, and therefore creating better treatments.

Chapter 11) Current prominent researchers in prosopagnosia

Research continues to develop our understanding of the condition with the aim to not only provide optimal treatment for individuals for the disorder, but to open doors to our understanding of face processing. There are currently a number of researchers who specialise in prosopagnosia, which are given below:

Bradley Duchaine

Bradley Duchaine is an associate professor of psychological and brain sciences at Dartmouth College. He has been at the College since 2010. Prior to this, he was a senior lecturer and a group leader lab at University College London. He was also a postdoctoral fellow at the Vision Sciences Lab at Harvard University.

Previous published work includes research looking into the inheritability of face recognition, and the connection between prosopagnosia and within-class object agnosia. His current research includes research on developmental prosopagnosia in children, the architecture of human face processing and investigations of the role and cortico-cortical interactions of the right occipital face area. The department regularly look for participants and so if you are interested in potentially taking part and are located in the

USA, the following link will take you Duchaine's page, which gives you more information about his work, and links to pages where you can mark your interest.

http://www.dartmouth.edu/~psych/people/faculty/duchaine.html

Ken Nakayama

Ken Nakayama has been in the department of psychology at Harvard University since 1990. Ken is interested in investigating the questions regarding how we see and has published a number of papers about prosopagnosia, including most recently "Face gender recognition in developmental prosopagnosia: Evidence for holistic processing and use of configural information" and "Processing of the mouth but not the eyes in developmental prosopagnosia". Ken often works together with Bradley Duchaine for his publications on the topic. Together, Bradley and Ken have a website at http://www.faceblind.org where you can find out more information about prosopagnosia. Visit Ken's profile page at the Harvard University site to find out more information about Ken's interests and his publications.

http://visionlab.harvard.edu/Members/Ken/nakayama.html

Sarah Bate

Dr Sarah Bate is a leading researcher in the centre for face processing disorders at Bournemouth University. Sarah aims to provide theoretical insights into the condition of prosopagnosia. She also researches towards a potential sub-classification. Sarah is currently researching the nature of face processing impairments in children and adults. She is focussing this research for both developmental and acquired prosopagnosia. She is also an Author of a book titled "Face Recognition and its Disorders". Visit her page at the University of Bournemouth website to find out more:

http://staffprofiles.bournemouth.ac.uk/display/sbate

Ashok Jansari

Dr Ashok Jansari is currently a researcher of prosopagnosia at the University of East London. He first attained his degree in Experimental Psychology from Kings College Cambridge. In 2011 he was awarded a 3 month Welcome funded Live Science residency at London's Science Museum where he was to conduct one of the largest studies in the world on face recognition. His previous papers include "Covert face recognition relies on affective valence in congenital prosopagnosia." and "The man who mistook his neuropsychologist for a popstar: when configural processing fails in selective prosopagnosia." Dr Jansari is also a member of the Experimental Psychology Society and the British Neuropsychological Society. Visit his page on the University of East London website to find out more:

http://www.uel.ac.uk/psychology/staff/ashokjansari/

Concluding comments

As more and more people are realizing their condition in these modern times, there is now a demand, more than ever, to further our understanding of the deficit mechanisms of prosopagnosia. In particular, as we have discovered that developmental prosopagnosia makes up most of the individuals who have this condition, research in the area of developmental prosopagnosia has become one of the main research areas in the field at the moment.

Other directions which further research could take us, is a sub-classification of the disorder. We have already seen the condition split into subtypes since it was first defined in 1947. We have also seen that this condition can manifest in a number of different ways within each of these sub-classifications. For example, in apperceptive prosopagnosia, individuals who cannot process a face in order to see it clearly, may see the face in a number of different ways. We have seen in this book a couple of case studies that demonstrate this. One of these cases observed an individual who saw faces as "skewed", another who saw faces as all the same with "hollowed out eyes". It is not yet clear why or how these various different types manifest. The potential of sub classification would also reflect in the furthering of our knowledge in face perception.

The current focus on developmental prosopagnosia will also help us to improve the current testing methods for the condition. According to researcher Gruter, diagnostic testing for this disorder may soon become a regular practise.

As we learn that the condition is more prevalent than previously anticipated, knowledge for this area of research has become more in demand. The result from furthering our knowledge of this disorder will also help us towards answering the biggest question in face processing – are the mechanisms for face processing domain specific? For the time being, the debate is still open.

Further reading

As mentioned throughout this book, the advances of our knowledge of face processing and facial recognition are still growing. There are various resources available, which are not only great for those wanting to find out more about prosopagnosia, but for those who would like to find out more about the condition for personal reasons. Maybe you want to find out where you can be tested for prosopagnosia? Or perhaps you know someone who could benefit from the test. Please see the various resources below for more information.

Books

Face Recognition and its Disorders by Dr Sarah Bate

This book is written by the researcher Dr Sarah Bate who is a researcher at the University of Bournemouth. This book examines the mechanics of face recognition disorders and provides discussion points on existing research. This book is particularly useful as literature to read if you are a student, as it was written with students in mind. However, this book provides an overview which will not only provide students with a clearer understanding of facial recognition, but other researchers will also find this a stimulating read.

The Man Who Mistook his Wife for a Hat by Oliver Sacks

If you are looking for a book written from a neurologist's perspective, but with some humour, this book is for you. This popular book was written by the neurologist Oliver Sacks, in which he describes some of his patients in some detail, who suffer from various neurological disorders. The book comprises of 24 essays, which are split into 4 sections. Each deals with various particular aspects of brain function. The title of the book is taken from one of these cases where the patient is suffering from prosopagnosia and in one meeting with his wife and Sacks; he mistook his wife for a hat!

You don't look like anyone I know – a true story of family, face blindness and forgiveness by Heather Sellers

This book is quite opposite to the above book written by Sacks, as it was written from a patient's perspective. The author, Heather Sellers, suffers from prosopagnosia, which in her case is associative prosopagnosia meaning that she cannot recognise faces that should be familiar to her. Sellers was completely in the dark about her condition growing up. The truth about her condition became apparent 20 years later when she took the man she would marry to meet her parents. It was then that she discovered the truth about her family and herself. In this uplifting memoir, the author communicates a truth about her journey of which the message conveys a strong sense of connection and love in a family that appears to be so broken. In the most heartbreaking and chaotic of families love may be seen and felt.

Face perception and prosopagnosia by Yunjo Lee

If you would like to read material that was written from a research perspective, then this book may be for you. This book contains reviews from recent scientific findings in face perception. Using various methods, this work presents findings of previous work and extends this onto an insight of the neural mechanisms in face processing.

Katherine B Leeland – face recognition: New Research

This is another book that is also written from a research perspective. Presenting the latest research within the field. When it comes to the latest knowledge in face processing, a lot of the time cases such as cases of prosopagnosia can help towards our understanding of facial recognition. This book isn't about prosopagnosia specifically; however it does provide the latest research in face recognition, which is related to the condition.

Understanding facial recognition difficulties in children – Nancy Mindick

If you are looking for a book with a breakdown of all the facts of brain blindness with a focus of the condition in children, this book is for you. Whether you are a teacher, a parent, a child psychologist or anyone else who would like to support the learning and development of children with prosopagnosia, this book may be what you are looking for. Nancy understands that people don't just want to know about details of the condition, which may be discussed between researchers, but it is a very real condition that is affecting children right now at school and at home. Nancy communicates details of the disorder, including an explanation of the different types, causes and characteristics of prosopagnosia. As well as a factual account of the disorder, she also provides the right information so that, for example, a teacher may be able to spot the condition in a child by looking out for the right signs. Recognition of this condition can greatly benefit their general learning and social development. Nancy also explores the various issues surrounding diagnosis and disclosure. She also includes management strategies, which will allow individuals to copy and support them whilst they learn to navigate social situations.

Face processing: Psychological, Neuropsychological and Applied perspectives by Graham Hole

This book is designed to provide a review of research, which aims to answer some of the big questions in face processing, such as, "How do face processing systems develop in children?" This book also provides a review from various perspectives, including a Psychological, Neurological and Applied perspective. This book is useful for students who may want to gain a wide understanding of our current knowledge in facial processing.

The official patient's sourcebook on Agnosia: A Revised and updated Directory for the Internet age by Icon Health Publications

This book contains a wealth of knowledge that is useful for individuals who have prosopagnosia. It is designed as a self help book so that those who are looking for more information regarding the condition can educate themselves with the facts. Given this perspective for the individual of the condition, it is also useful for those who are providing the diagnosis and support – the doctors, caregivers and health professionals. We all know that the vast amount of information there is currently available can make it a little overwhelming on where and how to get the right information. This book has attained all of its information from reliable resources, including peer-reviewed research, public and academic sources.

Face perception by Bruce and Young

Bruce and Young have helped develop and shape the field over a 30 year period, so if you are looking for a book that provides a reliable and comprehensive overview of face perception, this is a book you should read. It provides information that is accessible for students, as it is written in a clear manner, which makes it very useful for knowledge and research purposes for those new to the field. The way the book is laid out also allows for digestible content. Information is presented from a behavioural, neuropsychological and cognitive neuroscience approach.

Biology and Cognitive Development: The Case of Face Recognition by Mark H. Johnson

This book looks at cognitive development from a face recognition perspective. Whilst some research suggests that newborns are born with an innate system to detect faces, other studies suggest that infants are exposed to faces for months before they respond to them. The question of whether face processing is an acquired skill, or is part of an innate mechanism we are born with is the biggest question currently in the field of face perception. This book looks at both perspectives. This book is a great read for students who are interested in learning more about the debate.

Online resources

There is now a huge amount of material available online, where you can gain more information about the condition. The following are some of these websites, which are relevant and insightful to research in prosopagnosia today. Some of these websites also provide means to test yourself.

Face blind

http://www.faceblind.org

This website represents both research centres at Harvard University, the Department of Psychology and University College London, Institute of Cognitive Neuroscience. The website also speaks to visitors who may feel they suffer from the condition prosopagnosia and provide some free online tests that you are able to take right from your home. The information entered into the website, will also be used for research purposes. They also say that whilst these tests are useful, they are not perfect tests and that there may be those that are suffering with prosopagnosia who do well on these tests. If you do well on these tests and still feel as though you have prosopagnosia, it is advised that you contact them directly, as there are more extensive and thorough testing methods that take place at their labs. If lab testing is what you are looking for, fill out their online form to get in touch.

Trouble with faces

http://www.troublewithfaces.org/

This is a website that is dedicated to a number of researchers based at City University London, University College London and Kings College London who are trying to better understand how people recognise faces and understand expressions. In particular, they are interested in how these abilities can be disrupted in developmental prosopagnosia and alexithymia. Their website also calls out to individuals who may be sufferers of the condition for research on the condition. They are currently recruiting UK based prosopagnosic individuals for paid research studies.

Prosopagnosia at Bournemouth University

http://www.prosopagnosiaresearch.org/index/information

This is a website for the research group at Bournemouth University. Much of their work relies on the participation of both adults and children with face processing difficulties. They are always looking for volunteers and individuals are selected for studies following an assessment.

Yahoo Face blindness – Prosopagnosia group

http://groups.yahoo.com/neo/groups/faceblind/info

This is a popular online group, which welcomes discussions on prosopagnosia. Members include those with prosopagnosia themselves, friends, family members, researchers, counsellors, students and more. The group explores various topics including providing answers to general questions about prosopagnosia and living with prosopagnosia.

Headway Group

www.headway.org.uk/in-your-area.aspx

Headway is a charity designed to help and support individuals who have been affected by brain injury. There are various groups available in the UK, which are available to those who may have prosopagnosia as the result of7 brain damage. The various groups provide great support for individuals- including rehabilitation services, social re-integration, respite care and community outreach.

The London Face blind Group

http://www.monicazenonos.counselling.co.uk/

Monica Zenonos is a qualified counsellor and also a sufferer of developmental prosopagnosia. Monica has provided an opportunity for those with prosopagnosia to meet others who have the condition. This is done through a group that meet up several times a year.

References

Asaad, W, F., Rainger, G., & Miller, E, K., (2000). Task-specific neural activity in the primate prefrontal cortex. *Journal of Neurophysiology.*

Bodamer, J. (1947). Die Prosopagnosia. *Archiv Psychiatrische Nervenkrankheiten.*

Bradshaw, J.L., & Wallace, G. (1971). Models for the processing and identification of faces. *Perception & Psychophysics.*

Bruce, V., & Young, A, (1986) Understanding face recognition. *British Journal of Psychology.*

Bruce, V. (1998). Recognising Faces. *London: Lawrence Erlbaum Associates.*

Busey, A. (1998). Physical and psychological representations of faces: Evidence from morphing. *Psychological Science.*

Cecil, D. (1973). The Cecils of Hatfield House. *Cardinal, London.*

Choisser, B. Face Blind! http://www.choisser.com/faceblind/

De Renzi, E., Faglioni, P., Grossi, P., & Nichelli, P. (1991). Apperceptive and associative forms of prosopagnosia. *Cortex.*

Diamond, R., & Carey, S. (1986). Why faces are and are not special: An effect of expertise. *Journal of Experimental Psychology: General.*

Duchaine, B., Germine, L., Nakayama, K (2007). Family resemblance: Ten family members with prosopagnosia and within-class object agnosia. *Cognitive Neuropsychology.*

Duchaine, B, C., Weidenfeld, A. (2003). An evaluation of two commonly used tests of unfamiliar face recognition. *Neuropsychologia.*

Duchaine, B., Yovel, G., Butterworth, E., & Nakayama, K. (2006). Prosopagnosia as an impairment to face-specific mechanisms: Elimination of the alternative hypothesis in a developmental case. *Cognitive Nueropsychology.*

Junod, T (June/July 2013). A life so large. *Esquire magazine.*

Farah, M. J., Wilson, K., Drain, M., & Tanaka, J.N. (1998). What is special about face perception? *Psychological Review.*

Goodall, J. & Berman, P. L. (1999). Reason for Hope: A Spiritual Journey. *New York: Warner Books, Inc.*

Grüter T, Grüter M. (2008). An Underestimated Handicap: Congenital Prosopagnosia. *Geneva, Switzerland: EUPO course.*

Grüter T, Grüter M, Carbon CC. (2008). Neural and genetic foundations of face recognition and prosopagnosia. *Journal of Neuropsychology.*

Gruter, T., Kennerknecht, I., Welling, B., Wentzek, S., Horst, J., Edwards, S., Grueter, M., (2006). First report of prevalence of non-syndromic hereditary prosopagnosia (HPA). *Am J Med Genet.*

Haig, N.D. (1984). The effect of feature displacement on face recognition. *Perception.*

Hancock, P. J. B., Burton, A. M., & Bruce, V. (1996). Face processing: Human perception and principal components analysis. *Memory & Cognition.*

Headways. Prosopagnosia: Face blindness after brain injury.*https://www.headway.org.uk/Core/DownloadDoc.aspx?documentID=3053*

Haxby,J , V; Hoffman, E, A; Gobbini, M, I. (2002). Human neural systems for face recognition and social communication. *Biol. Psychiatry.*

Hubel, D, H., & Wiesel, T, N., (1959). Receptive fields of single neurons in the cat's striate cortex. *Journal of General Physiology.*

Itier, R, J., Taylor, M, J. (2004), N170 or N1? Spatiotemporal differences between object and faces processing using ERPs. *Cortex*.

Jacques, C. & Rossion, B. (2006). The speed of individual face categorization. *Psychological Science*.

Jiang, F., Blanz, V., O'Toole, A, J.(2007). The role of familiarity in three-dimensional view-transferability of face identity adaption. *Vision Research*.

Kanwisher, N. (2000). Domain specificity in face perception. *Nature Neuroscience*.

Leder, H., & Bruce, V. (1998). Local and relational aspects of face distinctiveness. *Q. J. Exp. Psychol.*

Leder, H., & Bruce, V. (2000). When inverted face are recognized. The role of configural information in face recognition, *Quarterly Journal of Experimental Psychology*.

Leopold, D,A. (2006). Norm-based face encoding by single neurons in the monkey inferotemporal cortex. *Nature*.

Matthews, M. L. (1978). Discrimination of Identi-kit construction of faces: Evidence for a dual-processing strategy. *Perception and Psychophysics*.

McKone, E., Kanwisher, N., Duchaine, B,C. (2007). Can generic expertise explain special processing for faces? *Trends Cogn Sci*.

Nunn, K. A Postma, P, & Pearson, R (2001). Developmental prosopagnosia, should it be taken at face value? *Neurocase.*

Pallis, C, A. (1955). Impaired identification of faces and places with agnosia for colors. *Journal of Neurology, Neurosurgery, and Psychiatry.*

Perrett, D, I., Rolls, E, T., & Caan, W. (2004), Visual neurons responsive to faces in the monkey temporal cortex. *Exp. Brain Res.*

Rolls, E, T., Baylis, G, C., Hasselmo, M, E., Nalwa, V., (1989). The effect of learning on the face selective responses of neurons in the cortex in the superior temporal sulcus on the monkey. *Exp. Brain Res.*

Sacks, O. (1985) The Man Who Mistook His Wife for a Hat and Other Clinical Tales. *New York: Touchstone.*

Schwaninger, A, Lobmaier, J. & Collishaw, S.M, (2002), Role of featural and configural information in familiar and unfamiliar face recognition. *Biologically Motivated computer vision.*

Schyns, P, G., Bonnar, L., & Gosselin, F. (2002). Show me the features! Understanding recognition from the use of visual information. *Psychological Science.*

Sergent, J. (1984). An investigation into component and configural processes underlying face recognition. *British Journal of Psychology.*

Shevelev, A., Lazareva, N, A., Sharaev, G, G., Novikova, R, A., Tikhomirova, S. (1999). Interrelation of tuning characteristics to bar, cross and corner in striate neurons. *Neuroscience.*

Tanaka, J,W., & Curran, T. (2001). A neural basis for expert object recognition. *Psychological Science.*

Tanaka, J, W., & Farah, M, J. (1993). Parts and wholes in face recognition. *Q J Exp. Psychol A.*

Tanaka, J. W., & Sengo, J. A. (1997). Features and their configuration in face recognotion. *Memory and Cognition.*

Transcript for Oliver Sacks on face blindness http://ttbook.org/book/transcript/transcript-oliver-sacks-facial-blindness

Valentine, T. (1988) Upside - Down Faces: A Review of the Effect of Inversion upon Face Recognition. *British Journal of Psychology.*

Wigan, A.L. (1844). The Duality of the Mind. *London: Longman.*

CPSIA information can be obtained at www.ICGtesting.com
Printed in the USA
LVOW04s2359231015

459506LV00041B/2250/P